KETO DIET QUICK

Fast and Easy Weight Loss Recipes for Every Day incl. Meal Prep and Diet Journal

Emily A. Hughes

TABLE OF CONTENTS

Welcome to

'Keto Diet Quick: Fast and Easy Weight Loss Recipes for Every Day incl. Meal Prep and Diet Journal'

!If you're reading this book, you've probably heard about the Keto diet. The diet is designed to encourage the consumption of low-carb, high-fat food.

'High-fat'- probably not be what you'd expect for weight loss, right?

Well throw your old ideas about weight loss away!

This book is designed to introduce you to the basics of the Keto diet by providing information, guidance, essential recipes, and a 14-day starter meal plan. We hope that in the coming pages you'll learn how the keto diet works, the fundamental rules, and the benefits it may have for your health, and for your life.

So, what is the keto diet?

The ketogenic, or 'keto', diet is a low-carb, high-fat diet that has been shown to have a positive impact upon weight loss and certain medical conditions. The aim of the diet is to move the body into the metabolic state of ketosis.

Ketosis differs from the automatic metabolic state because it burns fat for energy instead of glucose (carbohydrates). Through limiting carbohydrate intake, the body is forced to find an alternative energy source. The body responds to this need for energy by producing ketones, an acidic chemical body designed to break down fat molecules as an alternative energy source. Ketones will break down dietary fat and body fat, in order to provide a steady supply of fuel to your body. In general, the body will enter a stage of ketosis after 3-5 days when consuming less than 50g of carbohydrates per day.

This is why the keto diet is low-carb, high-fat – the restriction of carbohydrates forces your body into a metabolic state of ketosis, whilst the high proportion of fat serves to ensure you have enough of an alternative energy source. For this reason, the optimum fat intake is 70-80% of your overall calorific consumption.

Fat in the body is used to protect organs, provide insulation, and also stored for the evolutionary reason of alternative energy. Back when our ancestors were living off the land, ketosis was necessary in the times when food, and therefore glucose sources, was scarce. The keto diet therefore activates a natural, primal response to historical stimuli.

What benefits will you experience from adopting the keto diet?

Weight loss

Muscle maintenance

Improved skin condition, in particular the effects of acne

Appetite regulator and increased satiety

Reduced cravings for high carb foods

A lower risk of heart disease

Additional medical benefits:

Epilepsy and seizure management

Positive impact on nervous system diseases, such as Alzheimer's or Parkinson's

Management, or reversal, of Type 2 Diabetes

How can you monitor your ketosis?

Ketones can be measured in three ways; on your breath, in your urine, and in your blood. When monitoring your ketosis at home the easiest way to do so is through keto urine strips or a breath ketone analyser, both of which can be easily obtained online.

Ketones are present in the blood, and their levels are measured in mmol/l. For the most effective ketonic metabolism you will want your ketone levels to be between 1.5-3 mmo/l, however you will enter nutritional ketosis from 0.5 mmo/l, and hopefully reap the rewards of the diet from that level.

In addition to measuring your ketone blood levels, it is also possible to roughly measure your ketosis through your daily and sustained carbohydrate intake.

What are 'net carbs'?

You will hear the term 'net carbs' time and time again on your keto journey, but what does it actually mean, and how does it differ from carbohydrates in general?

Net carbs refer to the amount of carbohydrates that the body is capable of digesting- the ones that don't present themselves as fibre. Dietary fibre is essential to ensure a healthy gut and bowel, but it isn't digested or absorbed. Therefore, the carbs from fibre within a food do not count as part of your carbohydrate intake.

It's easy to calculate your net carbs when you understand this point. Take, for example, a large peach- roughly 175g.

The **total carbohydrates** within this peach is 17g
The **dietary fibre** within this peach is 3g
Therefore, the **net carbs** will be 17g – 3g = 14g

Remembering this simple formula will make your life a whole lot easier to keep track of your carbs.

There are roughly 3 levels of carbohydrate restrictions based on net carbs per day. These levels are in line with the definition that **a low carb diet is a consumption of less than 130g of carbohydrates per day, or 20% of energy from carbohydrates**. These levels can be understood as:

Ketogenic	<20 g/day	4% energy
Moderate low carb	20-50 g/day	4-10% energy
Max low carb	50-130 g/day	10-20% energy

What are 'macros'?

Macros, or macronutrients, is another term associated with the keto diet. Macros refer to where your calories are coming from, and therefore how to calculate the ideal keto plan for yourself.

The ideal macro ratio to initiate ketosis is understood to be:

70% of calories from *fat*	(9kcal/g)
25% of calories from ***protein***	(4kcal/g)
5% of calories from *carbohydrates*	(4kcal/g)

To figure out your individual daily macro requirements you must first ascertain your daily calorific needs- you can do this online with a caloric calculator app.

Caloric needs vary greatly dependent upon factors such as age, gender, current eight, goal weight, activity levels, etc., so it is best to take some time to work out what you individually need.

Keto diet tips and tricks for weight loss

Here are our top 5 tips and tricks that we've found useful for optimum weight loss on a keto diet:

❖ Don't starve yourself
❖ Low-carb doesn't mean restriction- quite the opposite! Restriction and denial will often end in bingeing because your body is so hungrily desperate

for energy. Stick to the meal plan and be sure to always eat 3 meals a day. Try to include adequate fat and protein in each meal.

❖ Drink plenty of water

❖ Hydration isn't only good for your skin, but it's also a way to avoid some of the 'keto flu' symptoms, and stave away hunger whilst your body adjusts. Try to drink at least 1 litre of water a day, and stick to water based drinks.

❖ Eat whole food

❖ A lot of packaged foods can be misleading with their portion sizing and nutritional breakdowns. Be sure to properly check packaging if you do buy ready-made foodstuff, but we highly recommend you stick to buying fresh, whole ingredients, and cooking for yourself. Studies show that cooking for oneself results in lower calorie consumption, and increased enjoyment!

❖ Eat slowly

❖ Food doesn't enter the stomach instantly- it takes around 5 minutes for your body to fully acknowledge what its eating. Eating slowly increases mindfulness, enjoyment, and allows you time to register fullness. Check if you're eating on hunger or emotions by taking your time and savouring your meal.

❖ Don't count calories

❖ Perhaps counterintuitive, but the high-fat nature of the keto diet means that calories can look high, and therefore put calorie-control dieters off. But there's more to weight loss than just a calorific deficit- it's quality rather than quantity. The method of keto is to provide your body with what it needs for optimum biological functioning, so the calories are used as efficiently as possible. Because of this, don't count calories; trust your body to work as it sees fit.

KETO FOOD GUIDE

The keto diet may appear restrictive, but once you get to know the basics, you'll soon realise there's a whole culinary adventure at your fingertips! We've provided a comprehensive list of what you can safely eat on a keto diet, and the higher carb foods that aren't recommended. Refer back to these lists if you're ever confused, fancy experimenting with creating your own recipes, or are heading out to the shops and need some guidance.

KETO STAPLES

Vegetables

❖ Artichokes
❖ Asparagus
❖ Aubergine
❖ Bell peppers
❖ Broccoli
❖ Brussel sprouts
❖ Butternut
❖ Cauliflower
❖ Celery
❖ Courgette
❖ Cucumber
❖ Green beans
❖ Kale
❖ Leeks
❖ Lettuce
❖ Mushrooms
❖ Onions
❖ Pickles
❖ Pumpkin
❖ Radish
❖ Rhubarb
❖ Shallots
❖ Tomatoes
❖ Turnips

Fruits

- Blackberries
- Blueberries
- Cranberries
- Currants
- Strawberries
- Lemons
- Limes
- Watermelon

Fats

- Avocado +oil
- Butter
- Cocoa butter
- Coconut + oil
- Ghee
- Lard
- Olives + oils
- Nuts + butters
- Seeds + oils

Meats and poultry

- Beef
- Game
- Lamb
- Pork including bacon and sausage
- Poultry including **eggs**
- Deli meats eg. hams
- Liver and organ meats

Seafood

- Fish particularly – bass, cod, halibut, salmon, sardines, trout, tuna
- Shellfish particularly – crab, lobster, oyster, mussels, shrimp

Dairy

Full fat and unsweetened versions of dairy products are key to the keto diet.

- ❖ Cheese all kinds
- ❖ Cottage cheese
- ❖ Cream cheese
- ❖ Double cream
- ❖ Sour cream
- ❖ Yoghurt particularly Greek

These foods form the basics of any keto diet, and as such keep your fridge and pantry stocked with them.

Below you will also find sugar and flour alternatives- useful for baking and sweet cravings:

Sugar

- ❖ Allulose
- ❖ Erythritol
- ❖ Stevia
- ❖ Xylitol

Flour

- ❖ Almond flour
- ❖ Coconut flour
- ❖ Flax seed
- ❖ Nut flours
- ❖ Pea and protein powders
- ❖ Psyllium husk powder

Foods to avoid

Grains

- Barley
- Corn
- Oats
- Pasta
- Quinoa
- Rice
- Rye
- Wheat
- the 'baked' section eg. bread, biscuits, cake, cookies, crackers, tacos, wraps

Fruits

- Apples
- Bananas
- Grapes
- Mango
- Pears
- Pineapples
- Stone fruits
- Juices
- Smoothies
- Dried fruits

Vegetables

- Beetroot
- Beans
- Celeriac
- Corn
- Potatoes
- Parsnips
- Peas
- Sweet potatoes

Legumes

- Beans
- baked, borlotti, black, cannellini, kidney, lima, mung, pinto, refried etc.

- ❖ Chickpeas
- ❖ Lentils

Sweetened and flavoured
- ❖ Alcohol
- ❖ Dairy
- ❖ Carbonated drinks
- ❖ Coffee based drinks
- ❖ Energy drinks
- ❖ Vitamin drinks
- ❖ Yoghurt

WARNING

When switching to the keto diet it can be common to experience some uncomfortable side-effects whilst your body transitions for one metabolic state to another. These symptoms should not continue for an extended period of time, and if they do it may be necessary to meet with your doctor and discuss whether the keto diet is suitable for you. These side effects are so common they have been nicknamed 'the keto flu'! We have listed some of the common side-effects you may experience below;

DISRUPTED SLEEP

Whilst in the long-term keto dieters report a better quality of sleep, initially you may experience some insomnia. This should resolve itself as your body adapts.

FATIGUE

As the body is forced to produce ketones as it never has before, you may experience some fatigue when transitioning. Once your body has adapted to ketone production this should subside.

LACK OF CONCENTRATION

As with above, your energy is directed towards ketone production in the initial stages of the keto diet. This may lead to a temporary lack of concentration.

CHANGE IN BOWEL MOVEMENTS

Constipation or diarrhoea is the most common side effect when switching to a keto diet. Ensuring you have adequate fibre intake and are consuming a varied diet with a range of nutrients; this uncomfortable side-effect should be gone in a week or so.

ORAL HEALTH

Ketones can be tested for in blood, urine, and breath. As your ketone levels increase, they may lead to a dry mouth and bad breath. The good news though, is that this side effect can easily be combatted by drinking plenty of water (and having some gum on hand).

As with any diet, it is necessary to transition slowly in order to give your body time to adjust. The keto diet is not here to further the myth of 'carbs are bad'; rather it uses a shift in metabolic functioning (done through the restriction of glucose) for specific health related results. Initially this diet should be undertaken with caution, and only continued for extended periods if medically advised.

There is also the risk of entering 'ketoacidosis' if the diet is not properly undertaken and monitored. Ketoacidosis is a build up of ketones, and a dangerous increase in the acidity of the blood- this is often the effect of diabetes, alcoholism, overactive thyroid disorders, excessive exercise, and starvation. Symptoms of ketoacidosis resemble those of the keto flu, but more severe, and with additional symptoms such as trouble breathing, stomach pains, and throwing up. If you feel you are experiencing these symptoms seek medical advice immediately.

BREAKFAST AND BRUNCH

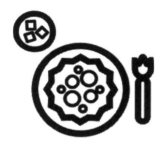

Granola

Using nuts and seeds instead of oats, this keto granola is great to make and store ahead of time. Have it as a quick breakfast with milk or yoghurt, or as a spicy, crunchy snack. We've provided a base below, but feel free to experiment with different nuts, seeds, and spices.

SERVES	3, 1c per serving
NET CARBS	8g
FIBER	12g
FAT	43g
PROTEIN	19g
KCAL	509

INGREDIENTS

- 150g // 1c almonds (chopped)
- 150g // 1c walnuts (chopped)
- 150g // 1c coconut flakes/chunks
- seed mix (2tbsp sesame + 2 tbsp flax + 2 tbsp chia)
- 1 ½ tsp cinnamon
- ½ tsp ground clove
- ½ tsp ground ginger
- 1 tsp vanilla extract
- pinch of salt
- 1 egg white (large)
- 120ml // 1/4c coconut oil (melted)

DIRECTIONS

1. Preheat your oven to 180C//350F, and line or grease a large flat pan
2. In a large mixing bowl combine all of your dry ingredients
3. In a separate bowl whisk the egg white until it begins to thicken, then stir in melted coconut oil. Add the egg white and melted coconut oil to your dry mix
4. Combine your wet and dry ingredients, stirring thoroughly to ensure everything is coated, then pour onto your prepared pan and flatten
5. Bake for 10 minutes, stir, and then return to the oven for a further 10-15 minutes. Cool the granola on the pan before transferring to an airtight container

The simplest Keto bread

Ready in under 2 minutes, this keto friendly bread really is simple! Great for any meal base or side, we've chosen to include it here as a quick and versatile way to start the day.

SERVES	4
NET CARBS	1g
FIBER	0.9g
FAT	8.4g
PROTEIN	4.0g
KCAL	98

INGREDIENTS

- 1 egg (large)
- 1 tbsp milk
- 1 tbsp olive/coconut oil
- 1 tbsp coconut flour (or the low carb flour of your choice)
- 1 tbsp almond or hazelnut flour (or another low carb flour of your choice)
- ¼ tsp baking powder
- pinch of salt

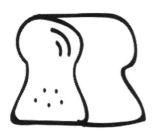

DIRECTIONS

1. Whisk together the egg, milk, and oil. Add in the flours, baking powder and salt, and stir to combine
2. Pour mix into a microwave safe mug, allowing the mixture room to rise
3. Microwave on high for 1 minute 30 seconds

TO TOAST

1. Remove your bread from the mug and cut into 1-1.5 cm slices
2. Fry the slices in a small oiled pan, turning until both sides are browned and crispy

Pancakes

Who said diets had to be boring?! Enjoy these low-carb pancakes free of guilt, and go wild with your toppings for a decadent morning delight.

SERVES	2
NET CARBS	4.1g
FIBER	1.3g
FAT	30.2g
PROTEIN	10.1g
KCAL	329

INGREDIENTS

- 120g // ½ c cream cheese
- 2 large eggs
- 30g // ¼ c low carb flour
- ½ tsp baking powder
- pinch of salt

DIRECTIONS

1. Place all ingredients into a blender and blend on high until a smooth batter forms- if you have no blender, whisk together the eggs and cream cheese before adding the remaining ingredients, and beating for thoroughly for 2 minutes until a smooth batter forms
2. Heat an oiled pan on high before adding your batter (2-3 tbsp should produce an average sized pancake). Cook until the bottom is browned, then flip and repeat on the other side
3. Repeat for the remaining batter- this recipe should produce 6 small pancakes.
4. Serve with sliced strawberries and cream, or bacon with syrup

Breggfast Wrap

This recipe substitutes the classic high-carb wrap for a high-protein alternative... eggs! Served here with ham and cheese, this recipe is great for breakfast, brunch, lunch, and dinner, and easily filled with whatever you may fancy.

SERVES	2
NET CARBS	4.4g
FIBER	0.5g
FAT	26.5g
PROTEIN	27.4g
KCAL	371

INGREDIENTS

- 4 eggs (large)
- 1 tbsp water
- 1 tsp cornflour
- pinch of salt
- oil (for frying)
- 85g // ¾ c shredded cheese (we used swiss, but cheddar, mozzarella, or emmental are tasty alternatives)
- 2 slices ham

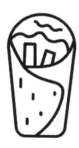

DIRECTIONS

1. Place the cornflour and water into a bowl and whisk until a paste forms, then add eggs and salt. Continue to whisk until it is fully combined

2. Heat 1 tsp of oil in a medium sized pan, sharing the oil to cover the whole pan

3. Add enough egg mixture to the pan to create a thin layer (about ½ c for a 12inch pan). Fry until the bottom and edges are browned, then flip and repeat. Add your ham and cheese- cover your pan with a lid for a minute if you like your cheese melted

4. Remove from pan and serve rolled and sliced

Sausage and Mushroom Frittata

Based on the classic fry up, this frittata takes the sausage, eggs, and mushroom triple threat to new heights! Cook up a batch to feed the family, or store in the fridge for a quick lunch during the bus week.

SERVES	6
NET CARBS	1g
FIBER	1g
FAT	26g
PROTEIN	20g
KCAL	333

INGREDIENTS

- 75g // 1c sliced mushrooms
- 300g // 2c sausage (chopped)
- 8 eggs (large)
- 1 garlic clove (crushed)
- salt and pepper as desired

DIRECTIONS

1. Before starting, oil a 10-inch dish and preheat oven to 200C//400F
2. Fry garlic, mushrooms, and sausage in a large pan until cooked and crispy, then transfer to the oiled dish
3. In another bowl whisk eggs until foamy, adding the salt and pepper for taste. Pour the eggs over the fried ingredients in the dish
4. Bake in the centre of the oven for 15-20 minutes. After this time has passed turn the oven off but leave the door ajar in order to rest the frittata for 5 minutes prior to removal and serving

Avocado, spinach and feta cheese frittata

A vegetarian alternative to our fry up frittata, the combination of avo, spinach, and feta is always a winner. You can even try swapping the feta for goats cheese to really make this dish something special.

SERVES	6
NET CARBS	3g
FIBER	3g
FAT	18g
PROTEIN	12g
KCAL	231

INGREDIENTS

- 1 bag // 4 c spinach
- ½ brown onion
- 8 eggs
- 1 tbsp milk
- 1 large avocado (diced)
- 120g // ¾ c feta cheese (crumbled)
- oil

DIRECTIONS

1. Before starting, oil a 10-inch dish and preheat oven to 200C//400F
2. Sautee onion and spinach in an oiled pan until the onion is soft and the spinach is wilted, then transfer them into the oiled dish
3. In another bowl whisk eggs until foamy, adding the salt and pepper for taste. Pour the eggs over the vegetables into the dish
4. Place into the oven and cook for 5 minutes, or until the edges have started to set. At this stage add the diced avocado, evenly sprinkling it over the dish
5. Cook for a further 5 minutes before crumbling the feta evenly over the dish. Having added both your feta and avocado cook for a further 5 minutes, or until the mixture is golden brown and cooked through
6. Allow to cool for a couple of minutes before serving

Green Smoothie

Start your day well with this spicy green smoothie! Packed full of iron and nutrients, this smoothie is great to fill up on whilst keeping macros low.

SERVES	2
NET CARBS	3g
FIBER	1g
FAT	8g
PROTEIN	1g
KCAL	82

INGREDIENTS

- 75ml // 1/3 c coconut milk
- 150ml // 2/3 c water
- 2 tbsp lime juice
- 170g // ¾ c spinach (preferably frozen)
- 1tbsp freshly grated ginger
- optional desiccated coconut to serve

DIRECTIONS

1. Place coconut milk, water, and spinach into blender and liquidise
2. Add lime juice and ginger to taste
3. Serve cold with a lime wedge and a sprinkle of desiccated coconut

Breakfast Bars

Why buy them when you can make them? Instead of going for the sweetened, packaged, high carb shop version, make these easy breakfast bars for the days when you need to be out the door pronto! Make a batch to store or freeze to ensure you never skip breakfast again.

SERVES	10
NET CARBS	3g
FIBER	3g
FAT	17g
PROTEIN	5g
KCAL	189

INGREDIENTS

- 🍽 40g // ½ c walnuts
- 🍽 40g // ½ c almonds
- 🍽 30g // ¼ c sesame seeds
- 🍽 30g // ¼ c sunflower seeds
- 🍽 2 tbsp flaxseed
- 🍽 5 tbsp shredded or desiccated coconut
- 🍽 30g // 1/8 c dark chocolate chips
- 🍽 3tbsp coconut oil
- 🍽 2tbsp tahini
- 🍽 1 egg (large)
- 🍽 1/2tsp salt
- 🍽 2tsp cinnamon

DIRECTIONS

1. Before starting, preheat the oven to 175C//350F and line a 7x11 baking dish

2. Place all ingredients into a blender and pulse until everything is finely chopped and combined. Spoon this mixture into your lined tin and flatten

3. Bake for 12-15 minutes, or until cooked and golden brown. Once cooked remove from the oven, and allow to cool before slicing

4. Keep in the fridge or an airtight container for up to 2 weeks, or freeze for up to 3 months

Banana Waffles

You can't generally have bananas on a keto diet, but these waffles are a sweet exception. Use a waffle iron for the iconic waffle shape, or fry for a pancake edition, this recipe is perfect for a weekend brunch treat.

SERVES	8
NET CARBS	4g
FIBER	2g
FAT	13g
PROTEIN	5g
KCAL	155

INGREDIENTS

- 1 banana (mashed)
- 4 eggs (medium/large)
- 100g // ¾ c almond flour
- 175ml // ¾ c coconut milk
- 1tbsp ground psyllium husk powder
- 1 tsp baking powder
- ½ tsp vanilla extract
- pinch of salt

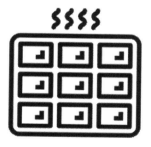

DIRECTIONS

1. Beat together eggs, coconut milk, vanilla extract, and mashed banana until smooth

2. In a separate bowl sieve the almond flour, psyllium husk powder, baking powder, and salt together, then fold this mix into your wet ingredients- be careful to keep as much air as possible. Allow the mixture to sit for 15-20 minutes

3. Using a waffle iron or frying pan, cook the mixture until golden brown

4. Serve with cream, butter, hazelnut spread, or whatever else takes your fancy!

Oatmeal

Comforting on a cold morning, this oatmeal is a way around the no-oat keto rule. Using absorbent seeds rather than starchy grains, have a warm bowl of this keto oatmeal when its gloomy outside. Experiment with spices and toppings to make it uniquely your own.

SERVES	1
NET CARBS	8g
FIBER	8g
FAT	61g
PROTEIN	10g
KCAL	615

INGREDIENTS

- 110ml // ½ c coconut or almond milk (unsweetened)
- 2 tsp flaxseed
- 2 tsp chia seeds
- 1 tsp sunflower seeds
- pinch of salt
- ½ tsp vanilla extract

DIRECTIONS

1. Heat the milk, sunflower seeds, flaxseeds and chia in a small saucepan. Bring the mixture to a boil before turning the heat to medium, and stirring in salt and vanilla extract to taste

2. Keep the mixture on the heat, stirring occasionally, until your desired consistency is reached

3. Transfer to a bowl and serve with a sprinkling of cinnamon, more seeds, or coconut cream.

LUNCH

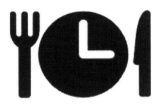

French Onion Soup

Go continental with our keto take on this French staple. Using cauliflower for a creamy texture, this low-calorie soup is a great lunch or starter. Serve with keto bread to mop up all the goodness!

SERVES	6
NET CARBS	7.1g
FIBER	2.8g
FAT	22.9
PROTEIN	8.8g
KCAL	274

INGREDIENTS

- 2 large brown onions (sliced)
- 450g // ½ large cauliflower head (chopped into florets)
- 4 cloves of garlic (whole)
- 4tbsp olive oil
- Salt and pepper to taste
- 960ml // 4 cups stock (vegetable or chicken work best)
- 240ml // 1c water
- 120g // 1c shredded cheese (gruyere works best with this classic)

DIRECTIONS

1. Before starting, preheat your oven to 170C//375F
2. Place sliced onion, cauliflower florets, garlic cloves, and oil in a roasting dish. Season with salt and pepper and toss everything to ensure the oil evenly coats the mix. Roast for 45 minutes, or until softened and browned
3. Whilst the vegetables are roasting heat your stock and water in a large pan
4. Once the vegetables are suitably roasted pour them into the pan and simmer for 10 minutes
5. The soup is ready to serve when all ingredients are softened and salt and pepper has been added to your liking. Serve topped with the shredded cheese

Broccoli and parmesan Fritters

Using broccoli for these fritters makes them low-carb and low-calorie, but deliciously filling! Paired with parmesan (or nutritional yeast) they're a fantastic vegetarian lunch to rustle up in less than 30 minutes.

SERVES	4
NET CARBS	5.3g
FIBER	4.9g
FAT	11.4g
PROTEIN	10.7g
KCAL	95

INGREDIENTS

- 🍽 350g // 1 medium broccoli head (350g)
- 🍽 4 eggs (large)
- 🍽 35g // 1/3c almond flour
- 🍽 50g // ½ c grated parmesan
- 🍽 1 tsp onion powder (packet onion soup works as an alternative)
- 🍽 1 garlic clove (minced)
- 🍽 chilli flakes, salt, and pepper to taste
- 🍽 1tbsp oil of choice to fry

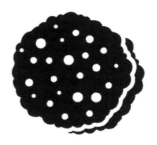

DIRECTIONS

1. Chop the broccoli into florets before placing them into a food processor. Pulse until the broccoli is finely chopped to a sand like consistency
2. Pour the blended broccoli onto a dishtowel or kitchen paper and leave for 10 minutes to remove any excess moisture
3. After the 10 minutes add all your ingredients in a large mixing bowl and stir thoroughly to ensure everything is combined. Leave to stand for a further 10 minutes before stirring once again. Divide the mixture into 4 and shape each ¼ into a fritter
4. Heat your oil in a large non-stick pan. Fry the fritters for about 4 minutes per side, making sure the bottom is cooked and crisp before flipping
5. Serve with salad and a chilli-yoghurt dip

Meatloaf

If you're looking for a protein hit then look no further than our keto meatloaf! Great for using up excess mince, this can be made ahead of time and is always a crowd pleaser.

SERVES	6
NET CARBS	4g
FIBER	2g
FAT	63g
PROTEIN	37g
KCAL	745

INGREDIENTS

- 1kg // 5c ground beef
- 2 eggs (medium)
- 1 ½ tbsp salt
- 3 tbsp seasoning (Italian herb mix works best, but try taco spice if you're feeling exotic)
- 1 ½ tbsp olive oil
- pesto mayonnaise (275ml // 1c mayo + 2tbsp green pesto) to serve

DIRECTIONS

1. Before starting, preheat your oven to 180C//350F and line a baking sheet
2. Combine beef, eggs, and seasoning in a large bowl- use your hands to ensure everything is combined
3. Form your beef mixture into a loaf shape and place on baking sheet. Rub olive oil and extra seasoning all over the loaf
4. Place in the centre of the oven and bake for 35-40 minutes. Once cooked, remove from the oven and set aside to rest for 10 minutes
5. Cut into slices and serve with leafy greens and pesto mayonnaise

Bunless Tuna Burgers

These bunless burgers look and taste gourmet but are incredibly easy and economical to make! A nice alternative to the average beef burger, serve these patties with a light salad or in a lettuce 'wrap'.

SERVES	8
NET CARBS	8g
FIBER	2g
FAT	79g
PROTEIN	39g
KCAL	911

INGREDIENTS

- 🍽 700g // 3c canned tuna 700g
- 🍽 80g // 1/3 c almond flour
- 🍽 2 medium green onions (finely chopped)
- 🍽 2tbsp chopped dill
- 🍽 zest of 1 lemon
- 🍽 1/2tsp salt
- 🍽 1/2tsp pepper
- 🍽 75ml // ¼ c mayonnaise (75ml)
- 🍽 1 egg (large)
- 🍽 1tbsp lemon juice
- 🍽 oil for frying

DIRECTIONS

1. Combine tuna, flour, egg, and mayonnaise in a large bowl, then add the onion, dill, lemon juice and zest, and season with salt and pepper. Stir again, making sure everything is thoroughly combined

2. Shape the mixture to form 8 patties, then leave them to rest in the fridge for 10 minutes

3. Heat oil in a large non-stick frying pan, then add your patties- cook for around 4 minutes each side, or until browned and crispy. Once fried place on a plate covered with a paper towel to remove any excess oil

4. Serve with leafy greens, lemon, and capers

Vegetarian protein kebabs

Based on a Mediterranean falafel but without the starchy chickpeas, try these protein-packed kebabs for a flavoursome lunch. Serve at a barbeque as kebabs, or shape into falafel balls for a Mediterranean power bowl, this mix has endless culinary possibilities.

SERVES	4
NET CARBS	16g
FIBER	14g
FAT	103g
PROTEIN	32g
KCAL	1124

INGREDIENTS

- 75g // ½ c sliced almonds
- 75g // ½ c pumpkin seeds
- 225g // 3c mushrooms sliced
- 125ml // ½ c oil (olive or coconut)
- 175ml // ¾ c pea protein powder
- 4tbsp chia seeds
- 1 tbsp diced garlic
- 1 tbsp coriander finely chopped
- 1 tsp ground cumin
- 1tsp turmeric
- 1tbsp onion powder
- 60ml // ¼ c water

- salt and pepper to taste

DIRECTIONS

1. Before starting, preheat oven to 170C//350F and grease a baking sheet
2. Toast almonds and pumpkin seeds in an unoiled frying pan for 2 minutes, then transfer to a food processor and pulse until they are finely chopped, but still have texture
3. Sautee mushrooms and garlic in 1tbsp of the oil until soft, then transfer cooked them and the remaining ingredients to the food processor. Blend once again, before pouring everything into a large bowl, and mixing by hand to ensure everything is fully combined
4. Let the mixture sit for 10 minutes, before shaping into balls or sausages
5. Bake in the preheated oven for 20 minutes, or until golden and crispy
6. Serve with a light salad and yoghurt tzatziki

Chicken Fajita bowl

Ditch the wrap and have your fajita as a power bowl instead! This spicy chicken salad has all the components of a Mexican fajita, but low-carb keto style.

SERVES	2
NET CARBS	9g
FIBER	11g
FAT	71g
PROTEIN	41g
KCAL	862

INGREDIENTS

- 1 head romaine lettuce
- 10 cherry tomatoes
- 1 avocado
- 2tbsp finely chopped coriander
- 1/2 yellow onion
- 1/2 green pepper
- 325g // 2c chicken thighs
- 1tbsp taco spice or tex-mex seasoning
- salt and pepper to taste
- 75g // 1c shredded cheese
- 125ml // ½ c sour cream

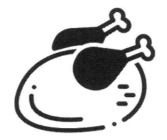

DIRECTIONS

1. Prepare your base by chopping lettuce, tomatoes, avocado, and dividing between 2 bowls

2. Cut the chicken into thin strips and fry in a medium pan with oil, salt, and pepper

3. Whilst the chicken fries, finely slice the onion and pepper. When the chicken is almost cooked through add the onion, pepper, and seasoning whilst stirring

4. Turn the heat to low and allow to cook for a few more minutes, before transferring the mixture to you prepared bowls. Top with the shredded cheese and sour cream

Chicken nuggets

Using cheese instead of breadcrumbs adds wonderful flavour to these chicken nuggets, and beans offer crunch and taste without the carbs of classic fries. Our twist on the takeaway classic with a Smokey BBQ sauce will delight children and adults of all ages.

SERVES	4
NET CARBS	6g
FIBER	2g
FAT	74g
PROTEIN	41g
KCAL	869

INGREDIENTS

- 500g//4c boneless chicken breast or thighs, cut into bite sized pieces
- 75g// 1/2c shredded parmesan cheese
- ½ tsp onion powder
- 1 egg (small)
- Salt and pepper to taste
- 2 tsp oil (we recommend coconut)
- BEAN FRIES
- 150g // 1c green beans trimmed
- 2tsp oil (we recommend coconut)
- BBQ DIPPING SAUCE
- 125ml // 2/3c mayonnaise
- 2 tsp tomato puree
- 1/2tsp smoked paprika
- 1/2tsp garlic powder
- Salt and pepper to taste

DIRECTIONS

1. Before starting, preheat your oven to 180C//350F and oil a medium baking tray
2. To create the nugget crumb, thoroughly combine the parmesan and onion powder in a medium mixing bowl
3. In a separate bowl whisk the egg until frothy, adding salt and pepper to season
4. Mix your chicken pieces into the egg and make sure that they are evenly coated with egg mixture
5. One at a time remove your chicken pieces from the egg mixture and coat in the nugget crumb, before shaking off any excess and placing evenly spaced on the baking tray. Repeat until all the chicken is used up
6. Bake the chicken in the oven for 15-20 minutes, or until crispy and cooked through. Turn halfway through baking.
7. Whilst the chicken is baking make the bean fries by heating the oil in a medium pan over a high heat. Once the oil is melted add the beans and fry for a few minutes so they are crispy- if fried for too long they will soften and wilt.
8. Make the dipping sauce by combining all the ingredients in a small bowl, adjusting spice measurements to taste
9. Once the chicken is cooked transfer to plates and serve with the bean fries and BBQ dipping sauce

DINNER

Keto Cauli Risotto

Low-carb risotto? Is that even possible? Well our keto cauli take shows that it is! Creamy and flavoursome, this risotto emulates the finer side of dining whilst remaining keto friendly. Remove the bacon and be sure to use vegetable stock for a vegetarian alternative.

SERVES	6
NET CARBS	4.7g
FIBER	1.9g
FAT	23.1g
PROTEIN	13.2g
KCAL	282

INGREDIENTS

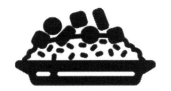

- 4 bacon rashers diced
- 60g // 2/3c mushrooms sliced
- white onion diced
- 3 garlic cloves
- 450g // 4c frozen cauliflower rice
- 160ml // 2/3 c veg or chicken stock
- 100g // 1c grated parmesan
- 160ml // 2/3 c double cream

DIRECTIONS

1. Fry the bacon until crispy on a medium heat in a large, deep frying pan, and once cooked transfer to a plate covered in paper towel
2. Sautee your onion, garlic and mushrooms in the same pan, using the bacon fat for oil. Once softened and browned, pour the stock and frozen cauliflower rice into the pan
3. Simmer for 5-10 minutes, or until the cauliflower has absorbed most of the stock, then stir in the parmesan and double cream. Continue to stir for 5 minutes to ensure everything is combined and cooked through
4. Remove from the heat and serve topped with your crispy bacon pieces, and extra parmesan if desired

Pizza

Higher protein and tastier than the normal cauliflower pizza, this keto spin on pizza is a cheese lovers heaven! Save money on a takeaway this Friday by making this keto pizza at home- it'll be done before the delivery would've arrived!

SERVES	2
NET CARBS	5g
FIBER	1g
FAT	90g
PROTEIN	53g
KCAL	1043

INGREDIENTS

BASE

- 🍽 4 eggs (large)
- 🍽 175g // 1 ½ c shredded cheese (we recommend mozzarella or provolone0

TOPPING

- 🍽 3tbsp pure tomato sauce
- 🍽 1tsp Italian herb mix
- 🍽 175g // 1 ½ c shredded cheese
- 🍽 toppings to your liking

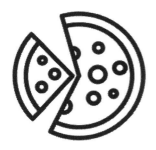

DIRECTIONS

1. Before starting, preheat your oven to 200C//400F and grease a baking tray
2. To make the pizza base combine the eggs and shredded cheese in a large bowl- the mixture should be wet, but still hold together
3. Spread and press the mixture onto your greased tray, shaping into a classic circle or as you please
4. Bake in your preheated oven for 10-15 minutes, or until the base is golden brown and crisp. Remove from the oven and allow to cool for 10 minutes
5. Once cooled, cover the base with tomato sauce and shredded cheese- at this point you can add extra toppings such as olives, pepperoni, vegetables etc.
6. Cook your pizza for a further 5-10 minutes. Allow the pizza to cool for a few minutes before cutting and serving

Keto bolognaise

As tasty as a classic bolognaise, we've used courgette 'zoodles' to make this recipe keto friendly. Keep your sauce simmering on the heat for as long as possible to get the rich, deep flavour of this Italian delicacy.

SERVES	4
NET CARBS	10g
FIBER	4g
FAT	31g
PROTEIN	26g
KCAL	425

INGREDIENTS

BOLOGNAISE

- 1/2 yellow onion, diced
- 2 garlic cloves minced
- 2 celery stalks, each about 20cm long
- 450g // 2 ½ c beef mince
- 1 heaped tbsp tomato puree
- 2tsp Worcester sauce
- 1tsp dried oregano
- 1tsp fresh or dried basil
- salt and pepper to taste

ZOODLES

- 3 medium courgette
- 1 tbsp oil

DIRECTIONS

1. Sautee finely chopped onion, garlic, and celery in a large pan on a high heat. Once browned and softened add the remaining ingredients and seasoning, making sure to stir and combine

2. Simmer on a low heat for at least 30 minutes, stirring regularly. If the sauce seems too thick at this point at 1tbsp of water and stir

3. Whilst the beef mixture simmers make your zoodles by using a spiralizer, mandolin, or peeler to cut courgette into ribbons. Alternatively, you can buy pre-spiralized courgette.

4. Heat the oil in a frying pan and flash fry the zoodles so they are softened, but maintaining some crunch

5. Transfer zoodles to a bowl and top with the bolognaise

Cheating Cheesy Chips

A British chip shop classic, using turnips instead of potatoes for your chips dramatically lowers the carb count and makes cheesy chips keto friendly. Serve as a main or a side to satiate your cravings for chips, or make it Mexican if you're looking for an alternative to nachos.

SERVES	4
NET CARBS	7.1g
FIBER	6.4g
FAT	17.6g
PROTEIN	4.7g
KCAL	212

INGREDIENTS

- 2/3 medium turnips
- ½ tsp garlic powder
- 1/2 tsp smoked paprika
- Salt and pepper to taste
- 3 tbsp oil of your choice (we recommend ghee or avocado oil)
- 60g // ½ c shredded cheese
- 4tbsp sour cream
- green onions to garnish

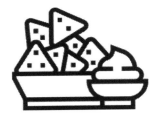

DIRECTIONS

1. Before starting, preheat your oven to 200C//400F
2. Peel your turnips and slice into fries- cutting them quite thin will ensure quick cooking and a crispy outcome
3. Transfer turnips to a baking tray and add the spices, seasoning, and oil- toss it all together to ensure the fries are evenly coated. Roast in the preheated oven for 35-40 minutes, or until cooked through, golden, and crispy
4. Top the fries with your shredded cheese (and any extras you may wish to add) before returning to the oven for a further 5 minutes to melt the cheese
5. Serve with a spoon of sour cream and sprinkling of green onions

Moroccan Fish Traybake

Any white fish will work to make this easy and flavoursome Moroccan traybake- a winning midweek dinner. Everything is cooked on one sheet pan so you can focus on the aromatic Moroccan flavours, and not be worrying about the washing up!

SERVES	2
NET CARBS	9.6g
FIBER	4.9g
FAT	33.7g
PROTEIN	30g
KCAL	475

INGREDIENTS

- 3tbsp harissa paste
- 1 lemon
- 2tbsp olive oil
- 2 white fish fillets (cod and haddock work best)
- 1 medium courgette
- 1 yellow pepper
- 1 red pepper
- 1/2 red onion
- 30g // ¼ c pitted black olives

DIRECTIONS

1. Before starting, preheat your oven to 200C//400F
2. Create the marinade by mixing the harissa paste, juice of ½ the lemon, a pinch of salt, and 2 tbsp of olive oil. Combine until it forms a loose paste
3. Use half of the marinade to coat your fish fillets, and set them aside to absorb the flavours
4. Chop the peppers, courgette, olives, and onion into slices, before placing into a roasting dish and tossing with the remaining marinade
5. Slice the remaining ½ of your lemon into 0.5cm rounds and place on top of your vegetable mixture
6. Roast for 15-20 minutes before placing the fish on top of your veg and cooking for a further 12-15 mins. The remaining cooking time is dependent upon the thickness of your fish fillets
7. Remove from the oven and serve immediately, topping with toasted pine nuts if desired.

Roasted tomato galette

Not quite a pizza, a quiche, or a pie, this rustic roasted tomato galette is a nod to southern French summers. The cheese-based dough makes this dinner low-carb and keto friendly, whilst supplying a healthy dose of protein and fats.

SERVES	6
NET CARBS	6.7g
FIBER	2.4g
FAT	29.3g
PROTEIN	22.6g
KCAL	381

INGREDIENTS

- DOUGH
- 100g //1c almond flour
- 170g //1 ½ c shredded mozzarella
- 1tbsp (heaped) cream cheese
- 1 egg (large)
- 1tsp onion powder
- ½ tsp garlic powder
- FILLING
- 250g // 1 ½ c cherry tomatoes
- 1 red onion
- 2tbsp fresh basil (chopped)
- 2 eggs (large)
- 2 tbsp ricotta cheese
- 60g // ½ c shredded mozzarella
- 1tbsp olive oil

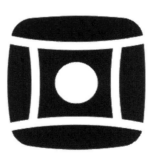

DIRECTIONS

1. Before starting, preheat your oven to 200C//400F , and line a baking tray with parchment paper
2. To make the dough heat the shredded mozzarella in the microwave. Do this by placing it in a microwave proof bowl, and heating then stirring at 20 second intervals until fully melted
3. Add the remaining ingredients and mix until it resembles a soft dough
4. Roll into a circle between two sheets of parchment paper- make sure the dough is evenly about 1/2cm thick. Leave the dough to rest
5. Whilst the dough rests start to make the filling- do this by whisking together the eggs and ricotta cheese until smooth, then add the shredded mozzarella, basil, and season with salt and pepper before beating to combine once again
6. Spoon the creamy mixture onto your dough base, being sure to leave a border of 2-3cm. Create a heightened crust by rolling this border inwards
7. Slice the red onion and sprinkle on top of the galette, then oil and add the tomatoes
8. Bake for 20-25 minutes, or until the crust is golden and crisp, and the filling is cooked through, but with a slight wobble in the middle.
9. Garnish with fresh basil leaves before serving

Butter chicken

Enjoy this Indian curry with cauliflower rice for a fragrant and filling dinner. Filling enough to feed the whole family and refined enough to serve at a keto friendly dinner party, butter chicken never loses its charm. The sauce can be made separately for a vegetarian alternative, or for any other dish needing some extra flavour.

SERVES	6
NET CARBS	7g
FIBER	3g
FAT	56g
PROTEIN	28g
KCAL	647

INGREDIENTS

- SAUCE
- 1 tomato chopped
- 1 yellow onion chopped
- 2tbsp freshly grated ginger
- 2 garlic cloves minced
- 1tbsp tomato paste
- 1tbsp garam masala spice
- 1 tsp chilli flakes (less if you don't like it spicy)
- 1tsp salt
- 175ml// ¾ c heavy whipping cream
- 900g // 7c boneless chicken thighs cut into bite sized pieces
- 4 tbsp butter or ghee
- Sliced coriander for garnish

DIRECTIONS

1. Create the sauce by placing all ingredients, except the cream, into a food processor and blending until a smooth paste is formed
2. Add the cream to this paste and blend once again until combined
3. Place your chopped chicken into a large bowl and pour the sauce over, stirring to ensure all chicken is covered. Leave this to marinate in the fridge for at least 30 minutes
4. After 30 minutes or more, remove the chicken from the sauce and heat 2tbsp of butter in a pan
5. Fry the chicken for 5 minutes, before pouring over the remaining sauce with the tbsp of butter. Turn the heat to low so the mixture can simmer for around 15 minutes, or until the chicken is cooked through
6. Add salt to taste before garnishing with coriander and serving

SNACKS AND SIDES

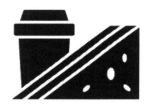

Essential cauliflower rice

This is just the basic, naked, no strings attached cauliflower rice recipe! This recipe is a staple for the keto diet and can easily be transformed into a main dish taste bud sensation with the addition of spices and vegetables, or it can be a simple side dish to compliment meat, fish, and vegetable mains.

SERVES	6
NET CARBS	13.4g
FIBER	5.4g
FAT	0.8g
PROTEIN	5.2g
KCAL	67

INGREDIENTS

- 700g // 2½ c cauliflower florets (around 1 large cauliflower head)

DIRECTION

1. Chop your cauliflower into florets, trying to leave as little stalk as possible
2. Transfer the florets into a food processor and pulse until broken down and sandy in texture- you may have to do this in batches dependent upon your food processor size. Be careful not to blend too much or you'll make cauliflower mash (also delicious)
3. Serve raw, or cook in 1tbsp of oil over a medium heat until softened

Creamed Spinach

A delicious side to add some iron and colour to a meal, this creamed spinach will upgrade any dish. This creamed spinach pairs fantastically with feta and chicken, and is a tasty stuffing for the latter.

SERVES	6
NET CARBS	2g
FIBER	1g
FAT	13g
PROTEIN	3g
KCAL	141

INGREDIENTS

- 🍽 3 tbsp butter
- 🍽 ½ onion diced
- 🍽 350g // 2c spinach
- 🍽 50g // ¼ c cream cheese
- 🍽 60ml // ¼ c double cream
- 🍽 1/4tsp garlic powder
- 🍽 Salt and pepper to taste
- 🍽 Grated parmesan to serve

DIRECTIONS

1. In a medium pan sauté your diced onion in 1tbsp of butter until softened and starting to brown- about 5 minutes
2. Add your spinach, cream cheese, double cream, garlic powder, and remaining 2tbsp of butter to the pan. Season with salt and pepper to taste
3. Cook on a low heat until the spinach is wilted, and the wet ingredients have combined to form a smooth and creamy sauce
4. Transfer to a dish and serve hot with a sprinkling of grated parmesan

Pesto egg salad

Serve this salad as a side or rustle it up as a quick and easy individual meal. The pesto dressing elevates this dish from plain to perfection!

SERVES	3
NET CARBS	2g
FIBER	1g
FAT	13g
PROTEIN	3g
KCAL	141

INGREDIENTS

- 3 hardboiled eggs (large)
- 300g // 1c cauliflower
- 1 medium leek
- 1tbsp oil

PESTO DRESSING

- 2tbsp green basil pesto
- 1 lemon, juice and zest
- 2 tbsp mayo
- Salt to taste

DIRECTIONS

1. Before starting, preheat your oven to 180C//350F, and oil a medium roasting dish

2. Cut the cauliflower into florets and slice the leek into 1-2cm rounds. Place in oiled roasting dish and toss together. Roast for 20-30 minutes or until softened and browned

3. Whilst the vegetables bake prepare the dressing by combing all the ingredients in a small bowl and stirring thoroughly

4. Assemble the salad. Use the vegetables as a base and place the sliced eggs on top. Drizzle dressing over

5. If serving as separate salads, add leafy greens for the base and top with a crumbling of feta for a light main meal

Hummus

Using courgette instead of chickpeas is the trick to creating a delicious keto hummus. This recipe can be adapted to your taste, and if you fancy add some avocado or roasted red pepper for something new. Serve as a dip, on bread, or as an addition to a meal.

SERVES	8 (1/4c)
NET CARBS	2.7g
FIBER	1.4g
FAT	14.9g
PROTEIN	2.2g
KCAL	152

INGREDIENTS

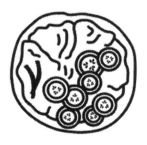

- 🍽 400g // 2 ½ c courgette cut into chunks for roasting
- 🍽 60ml // ¼ c olive oil
- 🍽 4tbsp tahini paste
- 🍽 2 garlic cloves minced
- 🍽 3tbsp lemon juice
- 🍽 Salt and pepper to taste
- 🍽 water as needed

DIRECTIONS

1. Preheat your oven to 180C//350F and place your courgette chunks in a medium roasting dish. Toss in tbsp of oil and season with salt and pepper.
2. Roast for 25 minutes, or until softened and browned
3. Once roasted, add the courgette and remaining ingredients (except the water) t a food processor, and blend until it is smooth in consistency. The hummus should be thick and hold its shape, but water can be added 1tbsp at a time if you desire a thinner consistency
4. Serve as a dip or accompaniment, topped with toasted sesame seeds and olive oil as a garnish

Pumpkin and Feta salad

It may be here as a side, but this pumpkin and feta salad is a lovely and colourful meal in its own right! So simple to make but flavoursome and filling, try this recipe for a light and summery meal.

SERVES	4
NET CARBS	7.1g
FIBER	1.2g
FAT	26.6g
PROTEIN	9.5g
KCAL	299

INGREDIENTS

- 🍽 300g // 1 ½ c pumpkin cubed
- 🍽 150g // 1c feta
- 🍽 Leafy greens such as rocket, spinach, or romaine lettuce
- 🍽 4tbsp olive oil
- 🍽 1tbsp balsamic vinegar

DIRECTIONS

1. Before starting, preheat your oven to 200C//400F.
2. Whilst the oven heats up peel and cube your pumpkin into bite sized pieces – the smaller your pieces the quicker the roasting time. Place these into a roasting tin and toss in 2tbsp of oil, plus salt and pepper to taste. Roast for 35-45 minutes, or until the pumpkin has darkened and softened.
3. Leave your pumpkin to cool, and in the meantime wash your leafy greens and mix the remaining 2 tbsp of olive oil with the balsamic to create a simple dressing
4. To serve layer the pumpkin on top of the greens and crumble the feta over. Drizzle with the balsamic dressing, and add pumpkin seeds or grated beetroot as an extra garnish if desired

Chocolate spread

This chocolate spread is the answer to any sweet cravings! Use it to smother your breakfast or have a spoon for a snack-enjoy our chocolate spread without any guilt and knowing that it's perfectly keto friendly

SERVES	10
NET CARBS	2g
FIBER	3g
FAT	28g
PROTEIN	4g
KCAL	271

INGREDIENTS

- 225g // 1 ½ c hazelnuts
- 100ml // 2/5c coconut oil
- 50g // ¼ c butter
- 3 ½ tbsp cocoa powder
- 2 tsp vanilla extract

DIRECTIONS

1. Dry fry your hazelnuts in a large pan to toast them. Watch them carefully as they burn easily, and remove from the heat immediately once they have turned a golden brown
2. Place the hazelnuts in a kitchen towel and rub vigorously- this will remove most of the skin
3. Transfer the hazelnuts to a food processor and blend with the remaining ingredients. The smoothness will depend on how long you blend them for, so check every 10 seconds until your spread has reached your desired consistency
4. Store in a jar in the fridge

Lava cake

Our keto meal plan may focus on your three meals a day, but don't let that stop you snacking on something sweet! Everyone deserves this gooey lava cake once in a while without having to worry about calories or carbs.

SERVES	4
NET CARBS	4g
FIBER	1g
FAT	16g
PROTEIN	4g
KCAL	180

INGREDIENTS

- 45g // ¼ c dark chocolate chips (min 70% cocoa solids)
- 3 tbsp butter (plus extra for greasing)
- ½ tsp vanilla extract
- 2 eggs

DIRECTIONS

1. Before starting, preheat your oven to 200C//400F, and grease 4 ramekins
2. Create a bain-marie by placing a glass bowl over a saucepan of boiling water- make sure the water does not touch the bottom of the bowl. Add chocolate chips and butter to bowl, and melt whilst stirring
3. Once melted set the chocolate mixture aside to cool slightly
4. Whilst the chocolate cools whisk together eggs and vanilla in a separate bowl until fluffy
5. Fold the chocolate into the eggs, being careful to keep in the air for a light batter
6. Pour the batter into the prepared ramekins and reduce oven temperature to 175C//350F. Place ramekins in the centre of the oven and bake for 4-7 minutes, checking regularly
7. Once the puddings are cooked remove from the oven and allow to cool slightly before serving

Carrot Cake Chia

The best thing about this carrot cake chia? It's a perfectly acceptable breakfast! Putting the flavour of carrot cake into a creamy sweet treat, this spicy chia jar is sure to leave you smiling.

SERVES	4
NET CARBS	6g
FIBER	6.5g
FAT	19.6g
PROTEIN	7.6g
KCAL	247

INGREDIENTS

- 5 tbsp chia seeds
- 360ml // 1½ c milk of your choice
- 2tsp vanilla extract
- 1 tsp ground cinnamon
- 1 tsp ground ginger
- ½ tsp nutmeg
- ½ tsp mixed spice
- 110g // 1c grated carrots
- 200g // 4/5c yoghurt (we recommend Greek or coconut)
- 60g // ½ c chopped pecans or walnuts

DIRECTIONS

1. Place chia seeds, spices, and milk into a bowl. Stir thoroughly to combine, and place in the fridge for at least 30 minutes to soak
2. After 30 minutes make sure the seeds have absorbed most of the liquid. Remove from the fridge and stir in the yoghurt and grated carrot
3. Split your chopped nuts between 4 glasses, and pour the chia mix on top. Add an extra sprinkling of nuts and grated carrot to serve

Fat Bombs- key lime edition

'Fat bombs' are a common keto treat, so we've added this key lime pie edition for a light and tangy version. Make and store a batch of these treats to keep cravings at bay- in fact, maybe make 2 batches, because these will be eaten up in no time!

SERVES	10
NET CARBS	2.2g
FIBER	2g
FAT	24.4g
PROTEIN	2.5g
KCAL	230

INGREDIENTS

- 🍽 240g //1c full fat cream cheese
- 🍽 125g // ½ c coconut butter
- 🍽 55g // ¼ c cocoa butter (if this is unavailable coconut oil can be substituted)
- 🍽 4tbsp coconut oil
- 🍽 60ml // ¼ c lime juice
- 🍽 2tbsp finely grated lime zest
- 🍽 40g // ¼ c low carb sweetener (we recommend erythritol)

DIRECTIONS

1. Start by beating together the cream cheese, coconut butter, cocoa butter and coconut oil until smooth and combined

2. Add the lime juice, zest, and sweetener, and beat again so the mix is smooth, but thick

3. Divide the mixture into 10 balls and place onto a parchment lined baking tray. Place in the freezer for 30 minutes to harden

4. After 30 minutes the balls can be removed and rolled in desiccated coconut for extra texture if desired. Keep in an airtight container in the fridge for a week, or in the freezer for 3 months

Classic cheesecake bars

Our keto take on the classic New York baked cheesecake, these cheesecake bars are as good as the original. We've provided the recipe for a light and creamy vanilla version, but feel free to add your own spin. This cheesecake also pairs well with our keto chocolate spread if you're looking for a crowd-pleaser!

SERVES	12
NET CARBS	5.5g
FIBER	1.9g
FAT	40.6g
PROTEIN	10g
KCAL	391

INGREDIENTS

BASE

- 🍽 200g //2c almond flour
- 🍽 6tbsp melted butter

FILLING

- 🍽 900g // 3½ c full fat cream cheese
- 🍽 100ml // ½ c double cream
- 🍽 40g // ¼ c erythritol, or alternative low-carb sweetener
- 🍽 15 drops liquid stevia, or alternative liquid sweetener
- 🍽 2tbsp arrowroot powder
- 🍽 1tbsp vanilla extract
- 🍽 3 tbsp lemon zest
- 🍽 2 large eggs

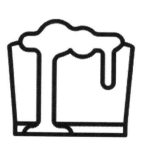

DIRECTIONS

1. Before starting, preheat your oven to 180C//350F, and line a 8x8 baking tin with parchment paper
2. Combine the almond flour and melted butter in a mixing bowl, kneading together until a smooth dough has formed. Press this into your prepared baking tin and bake for 10-15 minutes
3. Remove from the oven to cool, and increase oven temperature to 200C//400F
4. Prepare the filling by adding the cream cheese, erythritol, stevia, and arrowroot to a bowl, and mix using a handheld whisk
5. Still whisking, slowly pour the eggs into the mixture. Once the eggs have been combined, repeat the same procedure with the double cream, vanilla, and lemon zest. Pour this mixture over the base and level with a spoon
6. Cover with foil and bake for 35-45 minutes, removing the foil after 30 minutes. The cheesecake will be lightly browned with a slight wobble in the middle
7. Remove from the oven to cool for 10 minutes, before slicing into 12 pieces
8. Leave to cool further and set in the fridge for at least 5 hours (ideally overnight), before removing fully from the tin and enjoying

14 DAY KETO MEAL PLAN

This 14-day meal plan is designed to introduce you to the keto diet way of life! Comprising of all the recipes featured in the book thus far, and an extra bonus recipe per day, this meal plan is a way to ease into ketosis.

To follow this plan you don't yet have to have calculated your macros and ideal calorific intake- see this meal plan as a taster of the keto diet, and trust that in following it you will experience a gentle transition into a sustained low-carb diet.

All recipes can be easily adjusted to suit personalised servings, and we've made sure that all are stress free, from prep to the plate in less than 2 hours (including cooking).

So, go forth and feast with peace of mind and content satiation!

DAY 1

BREAKFAST: *Spiced pecan porridge*

SERVES	2
NET CARBS	4.6g
FIBER	10.5g
FAT	46.9 g
PROTEIN	13.3g
KCAL	532

INGREDIENTS

- 60ml // ¼ c coconut milk
- 180ml // ¾ c almond milk
- 4 tbsp almond butter (or the nut butter of your choice)
- 1tbsp coconut oil
- 4 tbsp chia seeds
- ½ tsp cinnamon
- ½ tsp nutmeg
- Salt to taste
- 30 g // ¼ c chopped pecans

DIRECTIONS

1. Place nut milks, nut butter, and coconut oil in a small saucepan and bring to a simmer
2. After simmering for 2-3 minutes add the chia seeds and spices and mix
3. Remove from the heat and allow to sit for 5-10 minutes to allow the mixture to thicken
4. If needed, reheat the porridge on a low heat for a couple of minutes, before pouring into bowls and serving. Top with the chopped pecans, and toasted coconut flakes if desired

LUNCH: *Bunless Tuna Burgers (See page 45)*
DINNER: *Cheating Cheesy Chips (See page 60)*

DAY 2

BREAKFAST: Breakfast Bar (See page 33)
LUNCHP: Salmon bowl with herby mayonnaise

SERVES	2
NET CARBS	4.6g
FIBER	6.3g
FAT	39.9g
PROTEIN	36g
KCAL	391

INGREDIENTS

- 200g // 1c large salmon fillet, flaked
- ½ an avocado
- 2 eggs, hard boiled
- 2 tbsp seeds (we recommend pumpkin)
- 2 tbsp mayo
- 1 tsp olive oil
- 1 tsp mixed herbs
- ½ lemon, juice and zest
- 1 garlic clove, minced
- leafy greens to serve

DIRECTIONS

1. To make your herby mayonnaise add olive oil, herbs, garlic, lemon juice and zest into a microwave proof bowl. Microwave for 10-20 seconds (this helps to develop the flavours). Remove and set aside to cool
2. Whilst the oil cools prepare your salad by layering greens, eggs, and avocado, and then sprinkling over the flaked salmon and seeds
3. Add your mayo to the oil and stir thoroughly to combine. Drizzle the herbed mayo over the salad and serve

DINNER: Keto bolognaise (See page 58)

DAY 3

BREAKFAST: *Granola with nut milk (See page 22)*
LUNCH: *Broccoli and Parmesan fritters (See page 41)*
DINNER: *Chicken, spinach, and artichoke cheese bake*

SERVES	6
NET CARBS	6.7g
FIBER	4.9g
FAT	31.5g
PROTEIN	43g
KCAL	391

INGREDIENTS

- 2 tbsp butter
- 1kg // 8c chicken thigh, cut into bite sized pieces
- 250g // 1 pack of frozen spinach, defrosted
- 1 tin of artichoke hearts
- 110g // ½ c mayonnaise
- 4 tbsp cream cheese
- 1 garlic clove, minced
- 1 tsp onion powder
- 1 tsp mixed herbs
- 50g // ½ c shredded cheese

DIRECTIONS

4. Before starting, preheat your oven to 180C//350F, and use the butter to grease a medium baking dish. Evenly spread the chicken in the dish

5. Finely chop the tinned artichoke and mix with the garlic. Add the mayo, cream cheese, and remaining spices. Stir thoroughly to combine

6. Place the defrosted spinach in a dishtowel and squeeze to get rid of any excess water. Place in a bowl and mix in half of your shredded cheese

7. Add the spinach mix into the mayo mix and stir until it is fully combined. Pour this over your chicken

8. Sprinkle the remaining cheese evenly over the dish before baking for 40-45 minutes. If the cheese starts to burn cover the dish with tin foil for the remaining time. Remove from the oven and serve

DAY 4

BREAKFAST: Pancakes (See page 26)
LUNCH: Easy egg salad avo

SERVES	2
NET CARBS	5g
FIBER	10.6g
FAT	56.8g
PROTEIN	16.5g
KCAL	617

INGREDIENTS

- 🍽 2 large avocados
- 🍽 4 eggs, hardboiled
- 🍽 6 tbsp mayo
- 🍽 ½ tsp smoked paprika
- 🍽 ½ tsp garlic flakes
- 🍽 Salt and pepper to taste
- 🍽 Optional spring onion, finely chopped

DIRECTIONS

1. Shell your hardboiled eggs and place in a bowl with the mayo, paprika, garlic, and seasoning. Mix with a fork, breaking up the eggs to create the texture of your liking
2. Halve the avocados and remove the stones. Scoop out some of the flesh, leaving roughly 1cm all the way around
3. Add the excess avocado to the egg mixture and combine
4. Serve by dividing the egg mixture between the avocado halves, and top with the optional spring onion if desired

DINNER: Pizza (See page 56)

DAY 5

BREAKFAST: Sausage and mushroom frittata (See page 29)
LUNCH: Feta and pumpkin salad (See page 75)
DINNER: Beef roll ups

SERVES	6
NET CARBS	9.2g
FIBER	2g
FAT	48.6g
PROTEIN	34g
KCAL	600

INGREDIENTS

- 500g // 4c ground beef
- 240ml // 1c tinned tomatoes or passata
- 2tbsp tomato paste
- 1tsp mixed herbs
- 1tsp dried basil
- 1tbsp dried oregano
- 2tsp garlic powder
- 2 cloves of garlic, minced
- 2 medium courgettes sliced into ribbons about 0.5cm thick

SAUCE

- 360g // 1 ½ c cream cheese
- 120ml // ½ c double cream
- 1 egg
- 240g // 2c grated mozzarella

DIRECTIONS

1. Preheat your oven to 180C//350F
2. In a large pan sauté the ground beef, garlic, and spices until browned. Add in the tinned tomatoes and puree, stirring thoroughly to combine. Simmer on a low heat for 10-15 minutes
3. Whilst the beef simmers create the cheese sauce. Using a handheld whisk beat your cream cheese to soften. Add in the double cream and egg, and continue mixing until a smooth sauce has formed
4. Prepare a medium baking dish by spreading a thin layer of sauce on the base. Lay out your courgette ribbons and place a spoonful or two of the beef on before rolling up. Place the roll upright in the baking dish
5. Repeat until all the beef has been used up. Sprinkle half of your cheese over the beef rolls, pour over the remaining sauce, and sprinkle the rest of the cheese over the dish
6. Bake for 30-40 minutes. Make sure the top is brown and crispy before removing from the oven and serving

DAY 6

BREAKFAST: Breggfast wrap (See page 27)
LUNCH: Cauliflower baked eggs

SERVES	2
NET CARBS	8.4g
FIBER	4.2g
FAT	26g
PROTEIN	20.3g
KCAL	349

INGREDIENTS

- 🍽 400g // 1 ¼ c cauliflower chopped
- 🍽 45g // ½ c grated parmesan
- 🍽 3tbsp double cream
- 🍽 3tbsp cream cheese
- 🍽 2 tsp cumin
- 🍽 2 eggs
- 🍽 Salt and pepper to taste
- 🍽 Optional 'the simplest keto bread'

DIRECTIONS

1. Boil the chopped cauliflower in salted water for 10 minutes, or until it is soft. Turn the oven on to 180C//350F to preheat.
2. Once boiled place the cauliflower, ¾ of the parmesan, cream cheese, double cream, cumin, and seasoning in a food processor. Blend until it forms a smooth and creamy consistency
3. Pour the cauliflower cream into a small roasting dish or ovenproof frying pan. Create two wells and crack in either egg. Sprinkle over the remaining parmesan
4. Bake for 10-15 minutes, or until the eggs are cooked through and firm to the touch
5. Eat as it is, or add a slice of 'the simplest keto bread' for dipping

DINNER: Moroccan fish traybake (See page 62)

DAY 7

BREAKFAST: *Strawberry chia pots*

SERVES	2
NET CARBS	7.5g
FIBER	4g
FAT	17.9g
PROTEIN	8.7g
KCAL	230

INGREDIENTS

- 2 tbsp chia seeds
- 120ml // ½ c nut milk (we recommend coconut)
- ½ tsp vanilla extract
- 1/8 tsp ground black pepper
- 75g // ½ c strawberries chopped
- 1tbsp water
- 120ml // ½c full-fat or coconut yoghurt

DIRECTIONS

1. In a small bowl combine the chia, milk, vanilla extract, and pepper. Stir to combine, then place in the fridge. Leave to soak for at least 20 minutes
2. Place the chopped strawberries and water into a small saucepan and heat until simmering. Leave for 5 minutes, or until the strawberries are soft, then use a fork to mash the strawberries until they resemble jam. Set aside to cool
3. Once soaked divide the chia mix between 4 jars. Divide the yoghurt between the 4 jars to layer and add a spoon of the strawberry mixture to each
4. Serve with additional strawberries if desired

LUNCH: Avo and feta cheese frittata (See page 30)
DINNER: Butter chicken (See page 66)

DAY 8

BREAKFAST: Green smoothie (See page 32)
LUNCH: Meatloaf (See page 43)
DINNER: Spanakopita pockets

SERVES	2
NET CARBS	5.3g
FIBER	5.4g
FAT	27.9g
PROTEIN	21.4g
KCAL	363

INGREDIENTS

- 85g // ¾ c shredded mozzarella
- 1 heaped tbsp cream cheese
- 4 tbsp flaxseed
- 85g // ½ c spinach, boiled and with extra moisture squeezed out
- 85g // ½ c feta

DIRECTIONS

1. Before starting, preheat the oven to 200C//400F, and line a baking tray with parchment paper
2. To make the dough mix together the cream cheese and mozzarella. In a microwave safe bowl melt the cheese mixture, stirring at 20 second intervals- it should take about 1 minute overall
3. Add the flaxseed to the melted cheese and stir. Once combined remove the dough from the bowl and knead until smooth. Roll the dough out onto the lined baking tray. Try and roll the dough about 0.5cm thick, and into a roughly rectangular shape
4. Add the cooked spinach and feta to the centre of the dough. Fold the dough to seal in the filling, smoothing together the edges to ensure it doesn't leak when cooking. For extra safety use a fork to prick a few holes in the dough
5. Place in the centre of the oven and bake for 15-20 minutes, or until firm, golden, and crispy. Allow to cool for a couple of minutes before cutting and serving

DAY 9

BREAKFAST: *French Toast*

SERVES	2
NET CARBS	3.3g
FIBER	0.9g
FAT	47.5g
PROTEIN	32.6g
KCAL	546

INGREDIENTS

- 1 loaf of 'The simplest keto bread', cut into 4 slices
- 2 eggs
- 2 tbsp full cream milk
- 1tsp of low carb sweetener (we recommend stevia or erythritol)
- ½ tsp cinnamon
- ½ tsp mixed spice
- salt to taste
- 2 tbsp oil for frying

DIRECTIONS

1. Having made your 'simplest keto bread loaf', lay the 4 slices on a plate
2. Place all ingredients but the bread and oil into a bowl and whisk to combine. Pour half the mix over one side of your bread, then flip and pour the remainder over
3. Heat your oil in a large frying pan on a high heat. Fry two of the soaked slices in the pan at a time, cooking for 1-2 minutes on each side to ensure all the egg mixture is fully cooked
4. Transfer to plates and serve with toppings of your choice

LUNCH: Chicken Fajita bowl (See page 49)
DINNER: Roasted Tomato Galette (See page 64)

DAY 10

BREAKFAST: *Keto bread with chocolate spread (See page 77)*
LUNCH: *Pesto egg salad (See page 71)*
DINNER: *Spicy sausage stuffed spaghetti squash*

SERVES	4
NET CARBS	16g
FIBER	5.8g
FAT	40.4g
PROTEIN	26.4g
KCAL	584

INGREDIENTS

- 🍽 2 small spaghetti squash
- 🍽 2 tbsp butter or ghee, melted
- 🍽 1 white onion, diced
- 🍽 450g // 3c chorizo sausage, sliced
- 🍽 1 tinned tomatoes
- 🍽 120g // 1c shredded cheese (we recommend strong cheddar)

DIRECTIONS

1. Preheat oven to 180C//350F. Slice the squashes in half and remove all seeds. Place skin down into a roasting dish and brush with 1tbsp of the melted oil. Season with salt and pepper before placing in the oven to roast for 25-30 minutes

2. Whilst the squash roast, heat the other 1tbsp of oil in a medium pan. Sautee the onion for a couple of minutes until it has begun to soften, then add in your sliced sausage

3. Once the sausage has browned slightly pour in the tinned tomatoes. Simmer for 5 minutes, then remove from the heat

4. As the sausage cools stir in the shredded cheese. Once the squash is softened and roasted remove it from the oven and divide the sausage mixture between the 4 halves

5. Grill for 5 minutes so the cheese has fully melted before serving

DAY 11

BREAKFAST: Banana Waffles (See page 35)
LUNCH: Mediterranean rice bowls

SERVES	4
NET CARBS	8.2g
FIBER	3.6g
FAT	34.4g
PROTEIN	19.3g
KCAL	442

INGREDIENTS

- 1 batch of cauliflower rice
- 1 small red onion, diced
- 2 cloves of garlic, minced
- 4 tsp red pesto
- 15g // 1/8 c sundried tomatoes
- 2tbsp fresh basil, sliced
- 1tsp dried rosemary
- 1tsp dried oregano
- 3tbsp olive oil
- 320g // 1 block of halloumi
- Optional lemon to garnish

DIRECTIONS

1. Heat a large frying pan. Add 1tbsp of olive oil, then sauté the onion and garlic until softened. Lower the heat before adding another 1tbsp oil, cauliflower rice, pesto, tomatoes, oregano, and rosemary. Heat for 3-5 minutes

2. Transfer rice to a bowl, adding the fresh basil by tossing the rice- not only will the basil be incorporated, but the rice will be fluffier and lighter

3. Heat the final 1tbsp of oil in the pan. Whilst it heats chop the halloumi into 12 even slices (3 slices per person). Fry the halloumi in batches, allowing 2 minutes per side to ensure the cheese is golden and crispy

4. Divide the rice between 4 plates and top with the halloumi slices. Serve with an optional lemon wedge

DINNER: Vegetarian protein kebabs (See page 47)

DAY 12

BREAKFAST: Oatmeal (See page 37)
LUNCH: Chicken nuggets (See page 51)
DINNER: Vegetable lasagne

SERVES	6
NET CARBS	9g
FIBER	5.4g
FAT	38g
PROTEIN	20.4g
KCAL	473

INGREDIENTS

- 2 medium aubergines
- 240ml // 1c marinara sauce
- 300g // 2c spinach, fresh (blanched) or frozen (defrosted)
- 2tbsp fresh basil, chopped
- 1tsp dried oregano
- 1tsp dried thyme
- 200g // 1 1/3 c feta
- 160 g // 1 ½ c mozzarella, grated (or alternative shredded cheese)
- 6 eggs
- 85g // 4 tbsp ghee
- Salt and pepper to season

DIRECTIONS

1. Before starting, preheat oven to 200C//400F. Slice aubergines into slices roughly 1cm thick and place evenly on a baking tray. Coat with 2 tbsp of the ghee, melted, and season. Place in the oven for 20 minutes to soften

2. Whilst the aubergine bakes heat a large frying pan on high with 2tbsp of ghee. Whisk together the eggs, oregano, and thyme in a large bowl. Using 1/6 of the egg mix at a time pour a thin layer into the frying pan. Cook for 1-2 minutes on either side before transferring to a plate. Repeat for the remaining eggs

3. Once the aubergine is removed from the oven reduce the temperature to 180C//350F. In a medium baking dish start layering your lasagne. Line the bottom of the dish with 2 of the egg rounds, spread a layer of marinara sauce, then a layer of roasted aubergine. Repeat this to create 3 layers, adding the spinach and feta after the aubergine for the top two layers

4. Spread the grated mozzarella over the top of your lasagne and place in the oven. Cook for 25-30 minutes, making sure the cheese top is crispy and golden

DAY 13

BREAKFAST: *Granola and yoghurt (See page 22)*
LUNCH: *French onion soup (See page 39)*
DINNER: *Lamb Koftas*

SERVES	4
NET CARBS	5.1g
FIBER	1.3g
FAT	32.6g
PROTEIN	27.9g
KCAL	429

INGREDIENTS

KOFTA

- 500g // 3 ½ c ground lamb
- ½ white onion, diced
- 1 garlic clove, minced
- 1 tbsp fresh coriander, chopped
- 1 tbsp fresh parsley, chopped,
- 1 tsp dried oregano
- 1 tbsp olive oil
- Salt and pepper to taste

RAITA

- 250g // 1c full fat yoghurt
- 1 large cucumber, cut into ribbons
- 2 tbsp fresh mint, chopped
- 1tsp garlic powder
- 1tbsp lemon juice
- ¼ tsp salt

DIRECTIONS

1. Place all 'kofta' ingredients except the oil into a large bowl. Using your hands mix everything together until fully combined. Divide the mixture into 8 and shape the mixture into sausages before skewering with metal or (soaked) wooden skewers

2. Heat the oil in a large pan on high heat and cook the koftas in 2 batches, turning every few minutes to prevent from burning. They should take around 10 minutes to cook

3. Whilst the koftas cook combine all the 'raita' ingredients in a small bowl. Be sure to toss it to coat all the cucumber ribbons

4. Serve the koftas with the raita, and a leafy side salad. Add the hummus from our 'snack and sides' to get an even more Mediterranean feeling!

DAY 14

BREAKFAST: Bulletproof Coffee

SERVES	1
NET CARBS	0
FIBER	0
FAT	25.2g
PROTEIN	0.4g
KCAL	221

INGREDIENTS

- 🍽 1 cup of coffee – home brewing is best, but instant coffee will still work
- 🍽 2tbsp butter or coconut oil
- 🍽 ½ tsp cinnamon
- 🍽 Optional dash of nut milk and/or low carb sweetener

DIRECTIONS

1. Melt your butter or coconut oil and cinnamon in a microwave safe mug until melted- work in 10 second intervals to avoid burning
2. Whilst stirring continuously, pour your coffee over the mixture
3. Add your optional nut milk or sweetener, and serve

LUNCH: Breggfast wrap (See page 27)
DINNER: Keto cauliflower risotto (See page 54)